60 Green Smoothies for Rapid Weight Loss

Quick And Simple Recipes For A Slim
Sexy Body

by FlatBelly Queens

Published in Great Britain by:

FlatBelly Queens
345 Old Street
London
EC1V 9LE

© Copyright 2016 – Flatbelly Queens

ISBN-13: {978-1533320247}
ISBN-10: {1533320241}

Table of Contents

Introduction: _____ 4

Chapter 1: Benefits of Juicing _____ 6

Chapter 2: Types of Juicers _____ 10

Chapter 3: The Benefits of Fruits & Vegetables
_____ 14

Chapter 4: Storing and Drinking Juices and
Smoothies _____ 19

Chapter 5: Recipes _____ 22

Conclusion: _____ 84

Introduction:

Sixty-eight percent of American adults are considered overweight or obese, with more than one-third falling in the obese category. Being overweight and unhealthy has become an epidemic in this country. If you are reading this book, you probably have struggled or are struggling with your weight.

The other issue with the normal diet of many people is that they don't get enough of the vitamins, minerals, and nutrients in their diet to help their body function effectively. Because of this, they often feel tired and sluggish, surviving on caffeine and hoping that an extra hour of sleep will make them feel better. But sleep cannot make up for lack of nutrients.

But there is hope! You can make positive changes to your diet, get healthier, and lose weight. This book will give you 60 smoothie and juice recipes that will help you get the nutrients you need in your diet and assist with your weight loss goals. Used as a replacement or a supplement to your meals, the recipes in this book are delicious, easy to make, and give you the nutrients you need to have more energy, fill you up, and help you lose weight.

You have the power to make a positive change in your life. You can eat better, get more energy, and feel great. You don't have to be another number in the growing obesity problem.

Chapter 1: Benefits of Juicing

Juicing has become very popular lately. The reason is obvious: it's really good for you. There are so many health benefits to juicing, and being aware of each one will help persuade you of the benefits of drinking many of your nutrients. Not only is it easy to do, it is very healthy. Seven health benefits of juicing include:

- Rapid Weight Loss: People who juice enhance

their weight loss. They are putting only healthy foods into their bodies, providing them with many nutrients they need, and cutting the calories they take in every day. By juicing, you are saturating your body with healthy foods high in nutritional content and cutting calories at the same time. This is an essential step to weight loss.

- Quicker Absorption of Nutrients with Less Digestion: When you juice or blend to make a smoothie, you are getting the benefits of the nutrients in fruits and vegetables without the need for your body to work overtime to digest the food. Because the food is already broken up, the nutrients are more easily absorbable, giving you their benefits without any added stress on your body.

- Getting a Daily Serving of Fruits and Vegetables: Everyone has heard how important it is to get in our fruits and vegetables, but how many people actually manage to get in five servings a day, as recommended? When you juice, however, it is easy to get many servings of the healthiest foods. Most juice or smoothie recipes have at least two servings of fruits and vegetables, and many listed in this book have more than that. One or two juices a day will give you all the fruits and vegetables you need in your diet.

And why are fruits and vegetables so important? They contain vital nutrients to keep yourself healthy. The vitamins, minerals, and phytonutrients can do such things as guard against cancer, cardiovascular disease, stroke, inflammatory diseases, and even protect against cellular damage. By drinking smoothies, you will be protecting your body against two of the biggest killers: cancer and cardiovascular disease.

- Strengthening the Immune System: Two vitamins are necessary for your immune system to work well: Vitamin A and Vitamin C. By juicing, you will be adding both these nutrients to your diet. Vitamin A builds the immune system, so you will get sick less often. Vitamin C does this also, and has the added benefit of being an antioxidant, which helps protect the cells in the immune system so they can work better. Your body needs both these nutrients to stay healthy.

- Increase in energy: Juicing has the natural benefit of improving your stores of energy. When you eat poorly, your body will feel sluggish. Since most people aren't getting the nutrients they need for their body to function well, adding green juices will automatically improve your energy level. You will be getting the nutrients you need for your body to function at its highest level. By juicing, you will feel better and may even be able to eliminate that caffeine habit! With greater stores of energy, you won't be tempted to reach for cup after cup of coffee.

- Supports Brain Health: A study conducted by Vanderbilt University in 2006 showed that drinking fruit and vegetable juices and smoothies at least three times a week cut the risk of people developing Alzheimer's disease. The nutritious chemicals in the brain help prevent cellular breakdown, which improves neurological health. In other words, juicing helps your brain stay strong and resilient and can help to fend off the ravages of old age.

With all these benefits, there's no reason not to juice. Juices can be used to supplement a meal or replace them. And by adding juices to your regular diet, you can reap the benefits from increasing your intake of fruits and vegetables for years to come.

Chapter 2: Types of Juicers

There are many types of juicer/blenders on the market, and it may be confusing to know which one to buy. Plus, with many different price points, you want to make sure you get something strong enough to handle the juicing you will be doing, yet affordable enough that it doesn't break your bank. Here, five different blender/juicers will be described in different price points.

- The Vitamix Blender is a very popular choice. It is a professional grade blender that has the capacity to chop, blend, puree, and even deal with ice cubes without a problem. They are even self-cleaning, which makes them easy to maintain. Many people love this blender. However, at a price tag starting at $299, with professional styles ranging into the $600 range, not everyone can afford this piece of equipment. It is durable and can withstand regular use, even with the most stubborn foods.

- The Ninja Professional Blender is another powerful blender with the capacity to crush ice without a problem. However, some people complain that the blade tends to become dull fairly quickly, which means you need to order a replacement one on a regular basis. However, at a price of just over $100, it is more affordable than some other blenders on the market, such as the Vitamix. Some people also complained about this blender being rather loud, which is bothersome to some people. But it works really well for the purposes of making smoothies.

- The Blendtec is advertised as the world's best blender on their website. They can range in price from $319 to over $1000 new, and are advertised as restaurant grade. Many people love this blender, but some have complained about the seal on the bottom of the container leaking, and the company has had to replace them sometimes. Otherwise, people love this blender for its capability to blend, crush, or puree anything. At the price tag, it should be able to do everything you need.

- The NutriBullet was designed specifically to make juices and smoothies. With a price tag at about $100, including travel mugs, it can be an economical way to start juicing at home. It blends things directly in the cups that you drink out of, saving some clean-up. The biggest complaint that some people have is that it does not do as well blending frozen fruits and seeds from strawberries and raspberries, which makes it less than ideal for completely smooth juices. Also, you can only make one serving at a time, since the cups it blends in are smaller than a regular blender. But it can be a good option for a making a single glass without too much difficulty at a small price.

- At $130, the Oster Chrome Blender is a reasonably-priced blender that power through ice and tough vegetables, which is necessary for smoothies. It's dishwasher safe and has a glass jar, which some people prefer. The Chrome blender is used in bars all over the world, and many people report being very happy with the power of this blender for the price.

Unfortunately, to blend ice and vegetables, you need a powerful blender and the $20 model at the local department store just won't cut it. Investing in a mid-priced blender or better will ensure juicing pleasure for many years to come. Any of the five above will work well for the purpose of juicing and making smoothies.

Chapter 3: The Benefits of Fruits & Vegetables

In this section, the health benefits of different fruits and vegetables regularly used in juicing will be described. These are the key nutrients in juicing and knowing their properties will help you pick with smoothie or juice you would like to make for a specific purpose.

- Kale: One of the healthiest leafy, green vegetables around, kale has many vitamins and minerals, has been shown help lower blood sugar levels in people with diabetes, help lower blood pressure, and reduce the risk of stroke. It also protects against the loss of muscle mass as we age and reduces the risk of formation of kidney stones. Because it contains a high amount of fiber, it can improve digestive health. Plus it has fiber, potassium, vitamin C and B6. It is a great, healthy vegetable used as the base of many green smoothies.

- Apples: Apples are full of fiber and vitamin C. It's a sweet, satisfying snack that is low in calories, so it helps with weight loss and can also help lower cholesterol. An apple a day, as the old adage goes, also helps reduce the risk of cardiovascular diseases. People who eat apples regularly also reduce their risk of diabetes, can prevent the formation of hemorrhoids, and may even prevent gallstones.

- Spinach: A dark, leafy green vegetable, spinach also acts as a base for many green smoothies. Along with all the vitamins and minerals it contains, it has been shown to lower the risk of cancer, lower blood pressure, control blood glucose levels in diabetics, and even help reduce the risk of developing asthma. It can improve bowel functioning and improve the health of skin and hair. It's also a great source of magnesium, which is an essential nutrient that improves energy, improves muscle functioning, and regulates many different functions in the body. Considering many people are magnesium deficient, this is an important nutrient to add to the body.

- Coconut Water: At 45 calories per cup, it's important to be careful about how much you drink. However, people have seen it as the new, natural sports drink. It can be great to drink after a light workout as it replaces potassium, which is lost through sweat and acts as an agent to increase hydration. It aids in weight loss, has very little fat, and can even help clear up skin blemishes. It has been used to ease digestion difficulties and to lower the recurrence of acid reflux. It can eve help reduce blood pressure. Plus, it can help you deal with leg cramps, which are often caused by a lack of potassium.

- Coconut Milk: A creamy base for many smoothies, coconut milk is high in fat content, but that is not necessarily a bad thing. Healthy fats can actually assist in weight loss. Coconut milk also has antifungal and antiviral properties, so it can boost your immune system and fight many common illnesses. Some research has shown that it also inhibits the growth of some cancers.

- Almond Milk: A great substitute for dairy milk, almond milk has many health benefits. It can help improve your vision, increase the chances of weight loss, help develop stronger bones and muscles, and help the kidney to function properly. Also, it can be used to help maintain a healthy blood pressure.

- Bananas: Bananas are used in many smoothie recipes and have a great many health benefits. They help prevent leg cramping due to their high potassium levels. The can help fight depression, help reduce swelling, aid weight loss, reduce your risk of type II diabetes, and even help lower blood pressure. They aid digestion, help prevent kidney cancer, build strong bones, improve your immune system functioning, and can help stabilize blood sugar between meals.

- Blueberries: Because of their high levels of vitamin K, they can help maintain healthy bones. They have been shown to lower blood pressure, help manage type I diabetes, help prevent many types of cancer, and aid in healthy digestion due to their fiber content. They can also help fight wrinkles.

Incorporating these items into your diet go a long way to improve your overall health and functioning.

Your immune system will function better, your digestive system will become more regular, you'll have more energy, and you'll feel healthier. And drinking smoothies is a great way to get more of them and have a delicious tasting drink or meal to boot!

Chapter 4: Storing and Drinking Juices and Smoothies

While drinking smoothies and juices are great for the diet, it isn't always convenient because they don't store well. A juice will stay for about 12 hours, while a smoothie will hold up well for about 24 hours. Left any longer than this in the refrigerator, and the smoothie separates and the fruit starts to spoil. There are certain things you can do to make them store for the day they are made, so you can make one in the morning and take it to work later.

First, store it in a glass container that has an airtight lid. Fill the container up to the top so that there is no air in the container, which could oxidize the nutrients in your smoothie. Also, to prevent oxidation, add a lemon to the juice or smoothie. It also adds a little bit more vitamin C to your drink to make it even healthier.

In general, the longer fruits and vegetables sit in the refrigerator, the more nutrients they lose. This is why you may not want to make smoothies ahead of time. If, for example, you are short for time in the morning, you can cut up your ingredients the night before and just mix them in the morning, saving many of their nutrients in the ingredients, but it won't take very much time.

Smoothies, however, can be frozen. A good tip is to freeze them in an ice cube tray, and when you want a smoothie, put the number of cubes you desire into a glass and allow them to thaw. They will be blended without the need to do anything else. Many people have tried this and love having smoothies available anytime they want.

Higher calorie smoothies are great for a meal replacement, especially those which contain coconut or almond milk, as they have all the nutrients necessary.

Lighter smoothies can be used as a snack between meals to stabilize blood sugar and to give you a jolt during the day.

To make your own smoothies, the basic proportions are as follows: 3 cups fruit to 2 cups leafy vegetables to 2 cups liquid base (such as water, coconut water or coconut milk). This is approximately a 2/3 to 1/3 ratio of fruits to vegetables. Feel free to experiment with the recipes below and your own combinations and see what you come up with.

Chapter 5: Recipes

This section contains recipes for many smoothies. All these smoothies follow a paleo diet and many are green, meaning they contain green leafy vegetables as a base. There are both high calorie and low calorie smoothies here. In most recipes, if it calls for coconut milk, you can replace it with coconut water or regular water to make it lighter, but it will change the consistency of the smoothie along with the nutritional content. Determine if you are supplementing a meal or replacing it and choose a recipe based on this.

Unless otherwise indicated, all you need to do is cut up the ingredients, add them to your blender, and mix until smooth. For green smoothies, blend the leafy vegetable and the liquid together first, then add the rest of the ingredients and blend again. Drink immediately for best results, or save a smoothie for up to 24 hours in the refrigerator.

Shamrock Green Smoothie (serves 2)

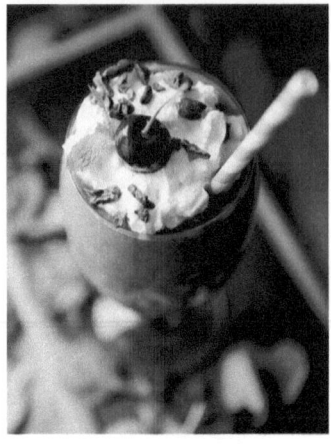

2 cups coconut milk, unsweetened
1 ½ cups fresh spinach
½ cup fresh mint leaves
2 bananas
4 medjool dates, pitted
1 teaspoon vanilla
Calories: 918, Protein: 10.2g, Fat 57.9g, Carbs: 125.3g, Vit. A: 65%, Vit. C: 44%, Calcium: 15%, Iron: 46%

Recovery Green Smoothie (serves 2)

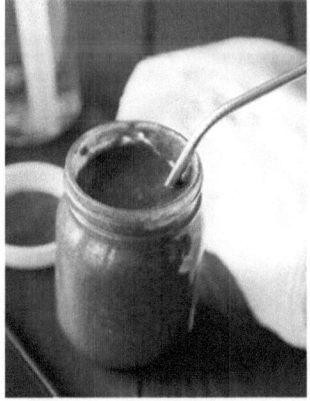

2 cups fresh kale
1 cup coconut water, unsweetened (or regular water)
1 orange, peeled
1 cup pineapple
1 cup blueberries
2 tablespoons chia seeds
Calories: 159, Protein: 3.8g, Fat .5g, Carbs: 39.1g, Vit. A: 211%, Vit. C: 300%, Calcium: 14%, Iron: 13%

Mint Green Smoothie (serves 2)

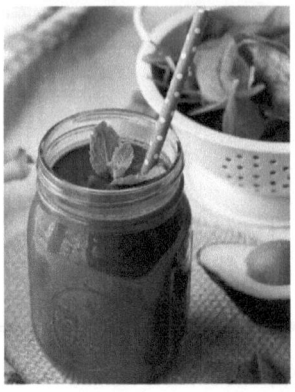

2 cups almond milk, unsweetened
1 ½ cups fresh spinach
½ cup fresh mint leaves
2 bananas
½ avocado
4 medjool dates, pitted
2 tablespoons cacao powder
Calories: 1027, Protein: 12.1g, Fat 68.7g, Carbs:
129.3g, Vit. A: 64%, Vit. C: 52%, Calcium: 16%,
Iron: 48%

Red Velvet Green Smoothie (serves 2)

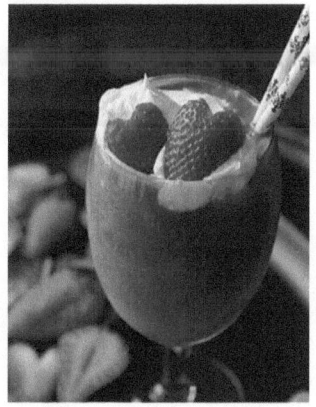

2 cups fresh spinach
2 cups coconut milk, unsweetened
2 cups strawberries
4 dates, pitted
¼ cup diced raw or cooked beets
1 tablespoon cacao powder
Calories: 667, Protein: 8.6g, Fat 58.4g, Carbs: 41.3g,
Vit. A: 57%, Vit. C: 168%, Calcium: 10%, Iron:
33%

Tropical Turmeric Green Smoothie (serves 2)

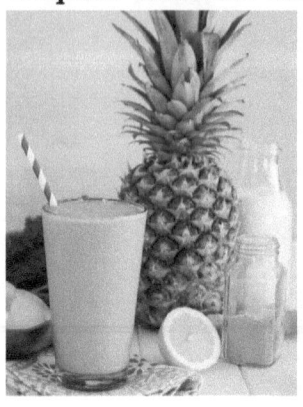

2 cups kale
2 cups coconut milk
2 cups pineapple
1 cup mango
Juice of ½ lemon
1 Tablespoon fresh ginger
¼ ground turmeric
Calories: 676, Protein: 8.6g, Fat 57.6g, Carbs: 43.9g,
Vit. A: 208%, Vit. C: 277%, Calcium: 15%, Iron:
32%

Citrus Beet Green Smoothie (serves 2)

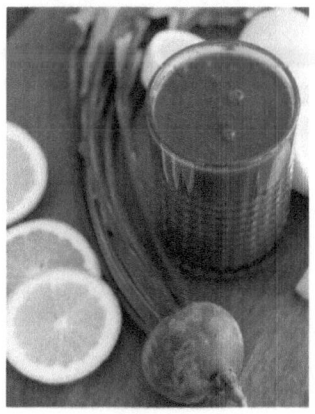

2 cups beet greens or chard
1 cup water
2 oranges, peeled
1 small raw beet, peeled and diced
Juice of ½ lemon
Calories: 115, Protein: 3.2g, Fat .4g, Carbs: 28g, Vit.
A: 53%, Vit. C: 184%, Calcium: 10%, Iron: 184%

Strawberry Banana Blueberry Juice (serves 2)

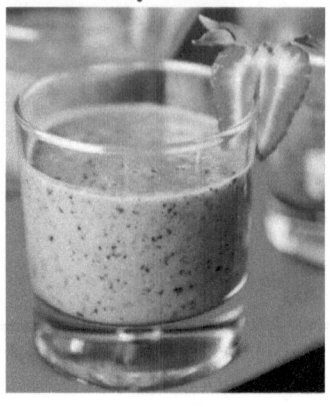

2 cups spinach, fresh
3⁄4 cup water
3⁄4 cup orange juice
1 cup strawberries
1 cup blueberries
2 bananas
Blend spinach, orange juice and water until
smooth. Next add the remaining fruits and blend
again.
Calories: 235, Protein: 4.1g, Fat 1.2g, Carbs: 57.5g,
Vit. A: 58%, Vit. C: 300%, Calcium: 5%, Iron: 22%

Beginner Juice (serves 2)

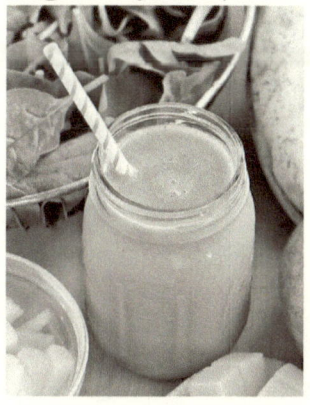

2 cups spinach, fresh
2 cups water
1 cup pineapple
1 cup mango
2 bananas
Calories: 225, Protein: 3.1g, Fat 0.9g, Carbs: 56.5g,
Vit. A: 75%, Vit C: 145%, Calcium: 6%, Iron: 8%

Pomegranate Citrus Drink (serves 2)

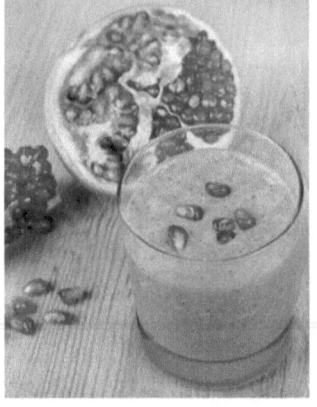

2 cups spinach, fresh
1 cup orange juice, fresh squeezed
1 cup water
1 cup pomegranate seeds
1 banana
Calories: 215, Protein: 3.3g, Fat 1.2g, Carbs: 515g,
Vit. A: 57%, Vit C: 210%, Calcium: 4%, Iron: 16%

Berry Cherry (serves 2)

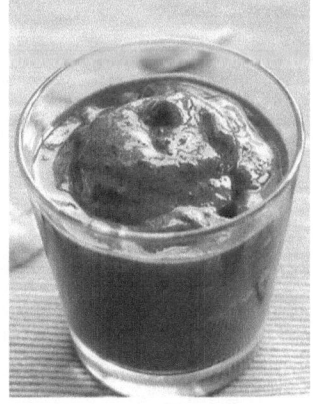

2 cups spinach, fresh
2 cups water
1 cup cherries, pitted
1 cup mixed berries
1 banana
Calories: 142, Protein: 2.1g, Fat 0.6g, Carbs: 33.4g,
Vit. A: 59%, Vit C: 50%, Calcium: 5%, Iron: 8%

Skin Cleanse Drink (serves 2)

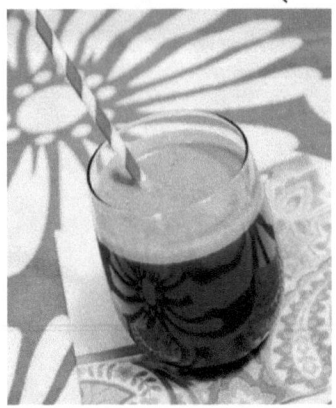

2 cups spinach, fresh
2 cups coconut water
2 cups pineapple
1 avocado
Calories: 340, Protein: 3.7g, Fat 19.9g, Carbs: 42.9g,
Vit. A: 61%, Vit C: 338%, Calcium: 9%, Iron: 11%

Free Radical Fighting Smoothie (serves 2)

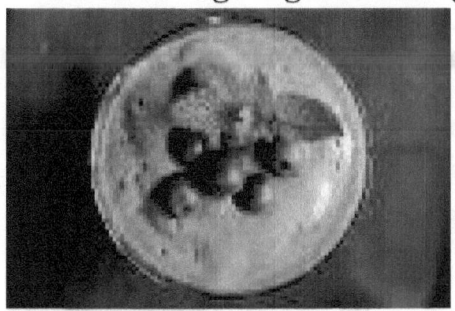

2 cups spinach, fresh
1 sprig mint, fresh
1 cup water, optional
2 cups cantaloupe, ripe and rind removed
1/2 cup blueberries
1 apple
1/2 lime, fresh squeezed
Blend spinach, mint leaf and ripe cantaloupe until smooth. You do not need to add a liquid-base to this recipe because of the high water content in ripe cantaloupes. Next add the remaining fruits and blend again.
Calories: 128, Protein: 2.7g, Fat 0.7g, Carbs: 31.6g, Vit. A: 162%, Vit C: 131%, Calcium: 5%, Iron: 11%

Sweet Potato Smoothie (serves 2)

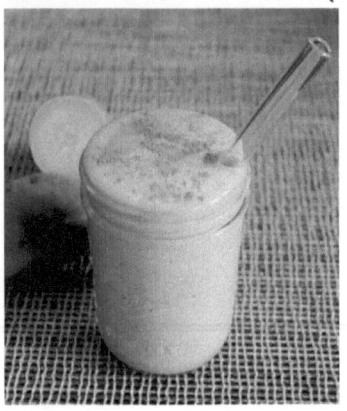

2 cups spinach, fresh
2 cups almond milk, unsweetened
1/4 cup water
1 cup sweet potato*
2 cups mango
1 tsp ground cinnamon
1 tsp ground nutmeg
Blend spinach, almond milk and water until
smooth. Next add the remaining fruits and blend
again. * Bake sweet potato at 400 degrees for 45
minutes. Then chill in fridge until ready to use. Use
at least one frozen fruit to make the green
smoothie cold.
Calories: 803, Protein: 9.5g, Fat 58.5g, Carbs: 71.8g,
Vit. A: 96%, Vit C: 175%, Calcium: 11%, Iron:
48%

Spinach Orange Smoothie (serves 1)

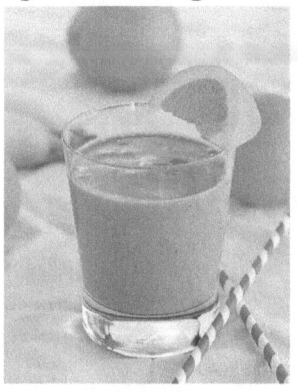

1 navel orange, peeled
1/2 banana, peeled
1 cup tightly packed organic spinach
1/4 cup coconut water, adjusted as desired
1 tablespoon hemp seeds, optional
A few cubes of ice
Calories: 188, Protein: 5.7g, Fat 4.0g, Carbs: 36.7g,
Vit. A: 65%, Vit C: 186%, Calcium: 11%, Iron:
11%

Ginger-Orange Green Smoothie (serves 2)

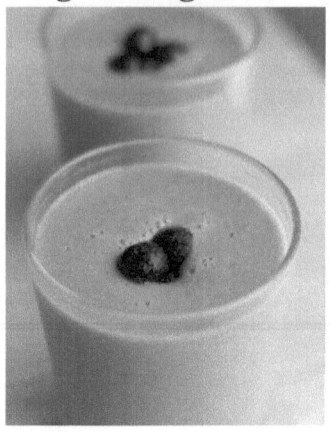

1 1/2 cups filtered water
4 generous handfuls fresh spinach
4 romaine leaves (optional)
2 navel oranges
2 ripe bananas
1"-2" knob of fresh ginger
1 cucumber (optional) peel if not organic
Calories: 229, Protein: 5.8g, Fat 1.0g, Carbs: 56.5g,
Vit. A: 125%, Vit C: 216%, Calcium: 16%, Iron:
16%

Emerald Kale & Mango Smoothie (serves 2)

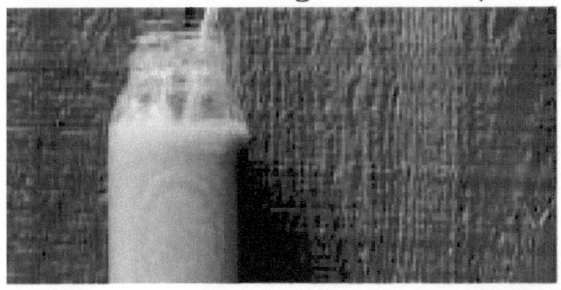

1 mango, peeled, diced, stone removed (keep refrigerated prior to using)
2 cups fresh kale – 2 large leaves, stem removed, leaves torn and washed
1/2 lime, juice only
1 kiwifruit, peeled and diced
1 cup cold coconut milk
Calories: 405, Protein: 5.7g, Fat 29.1g, Carbs: 36.8g, Vit. A: 222%, Vit C: 246%, Calcium: 13%, Iron: 18%

Almost Pina Colada (serves 2)

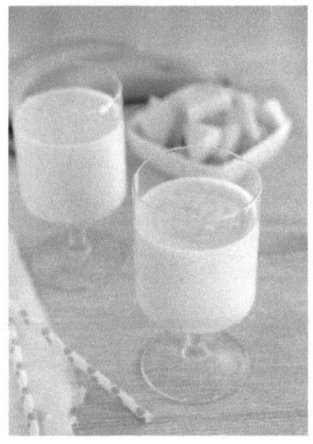

1 cup pineapple juice, fresh or with no added sugar
1 cup coconut milk
1/2 lime, juice only
1 banana
A few cubes of ice
Calories: 395, Protein: 3.8g, Fat 28.9g, Carbs: 36.2g,
Vit. A: 1%, Vit C: 35%, Calcium: 4%, Iron: 14%

Blueberry Acai Smoothie (serves 2)

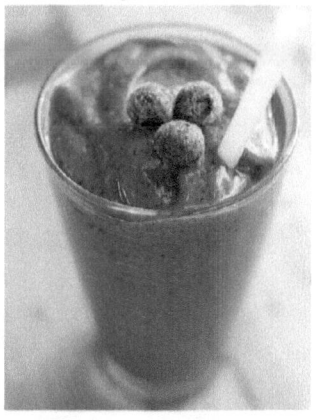

1 cup coconut milk
1 1/2 frozen bananas
1 cup frozen blueberries
1 cup frozen strawberries
1 cup acai juice
3/4 cup ice
Calories: 463, Protein: 4.3g, Fat 29.6g, Carbs: 53.2g,
Vit. A: 2%, Vit C: 117%, Calcium: 6%, Iron: 21%

Blueberry Beetroot Smoothie (serves 2)

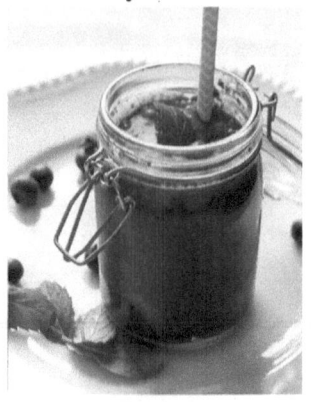

1 cup coconut milk
2/3 cup frozen blueberries
1 medium beetroot, peeled and grated (including the juice)
1 tbsp. lime juice
1/2 cup ice cubes or crushed ice
Calories: 328, Protein: 4.0g, Fat 28.9g, Carbs: 19.3g, Vit. A: 0%, Vit C: 25%, Calcium: 3%, Iron: 17%

Parsley Pear Green Smoothie (serves 4)

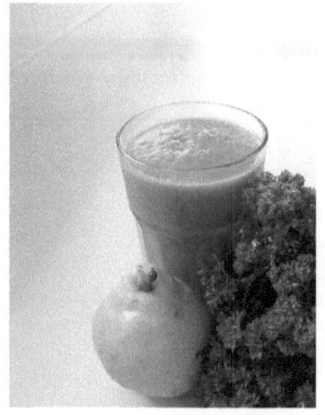

1 small bunch parsley
½ med avocado
1 nashi pear (aka Asian pear or apple pear)
1 pear
1 Royal Gala apple
1 Granny Smith apple
2 med plums
6 med bananas
1 cup water
1 cup ice (200g)
Calories: 296, Protein: 3.0g, Fat 5.8g, Carbs: 65.5g,
Vit. A: 7%, Vit C: 46%, Calcium: 2%, Iron: 6%

Heart Healthy Red Smoothie (serves 2)

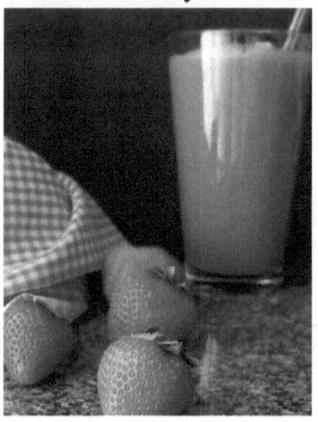

1 cup chopped red cabbage
1/2 red bell pepper
1 roma tomato
5 medium strawberries
1/2 cup raspberries
8 oz. cold water
1 ice cube [optional]
Calories: 64, Protein: 2.3g, Fat 0.7g, Carbs: 14.3g,
Vit. A: 20%, Vit C: 178%, Calcium: 3%, Iron: 15%

Cherry and Kale Smoothie (serves 2)

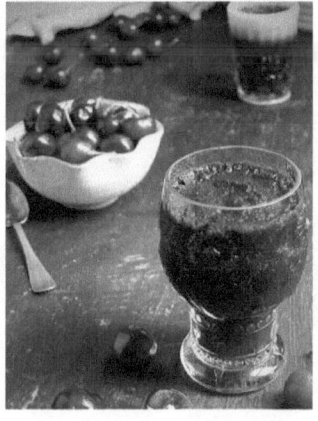

1 cup of fresh or frozen cherries, remove pits
1 cup of fresh squeezed orange juice
1 cup of kale leaves, chopped
2 tbs. hemp seed
1 tbs. raw coconut oil
1 cup of ice
Calories: 210, Protein: 5.1g, Fat 10.8g, Carbs: 25.8g,
Vit. A: 116%, Vit C: 69%, Calcium: 6%, Iron: 10%

Paleo Peach Coconut Smoothie (serves 2)

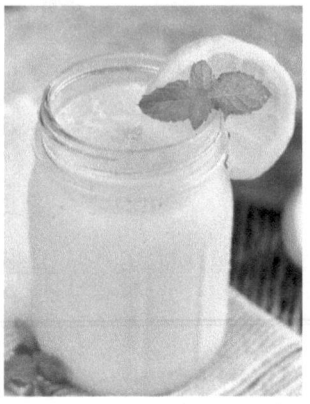

1 cup full fat coconut milk, chilled
1 cup ice
2 large fresh peaches, peeled and cut into chunks
Fresh lemon zest, to taste
Calories: 84, Protein: 1.4g, Fat 2.6g, Carbs: 16g, Vit.
A: 15%, Vit C: 17%, Calcium: 6%, Iron: 4%

Avocado Banana Recipe (Serves 2)

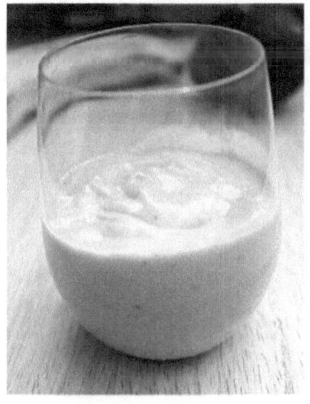

1 avocado, pitted
1 banana
1/3 cup spinach
1/4-1/2 cup water
Calories: 259, Protein: 2.7g, Fat 19.8g, Carbs: 22.3g,
Vit. A: 13%, Vit C: 28%, Calcium: 2%, Iron: 5%

Fall Harvest Green Smoothie (serves 2)

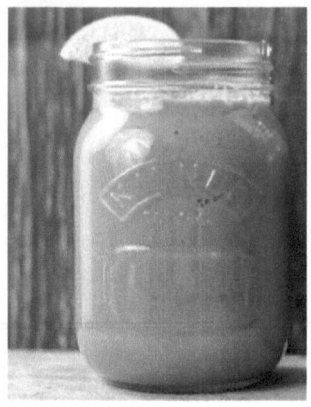

1 Apple
1 Orange
1/2 Lime – Peeled
1 Ginger (Frozen)
2 C. Spinach
1 C. Almond Milk
1 C. Ice Cubes
Grate the frozen ginger. Peel the lemon. Remove
the apple core. Blend it!
Calories: 379, Protein: 4.8g, Fat 29g, Carbs: 33g,
Vit. A: 61%, Vit C: 121%, Calcium: 10%, Iron: 19%

Pumpkin-Cranberry Smoothie (serves 2)

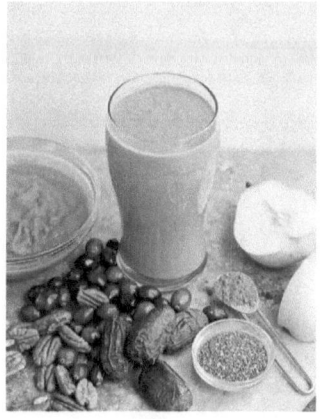

1 cup coconut milk
½ cup fresh pumpkin puree
¼ cup frozen fresh cranberries (raspberries would work in a pinch)
¼ cup raw 1 small apple, chunked
½ orange, peeled
2 tablespoons coconut cream (the fat atop a full-fat coconut milk can) or coconut butter
¾ teaspoon cinnamon
Calories: 521, Protein: 7.9g, Fat 42.1g, Carbs: 35.6g, Vit. A: 193%, Vit C: 67%, Calcium: 8%, Iron: 30%

Paleo Strawberries & "Cream" Smoothie (serves 2)

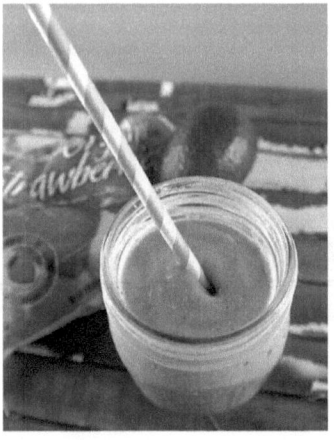

1 cup frozen strawberries (not thawed)
1 tbs. raw cashews
1 medium ripe avocado, peeled, cored and diced
1 cup non-dairy milk or water
1 tbs. raw honey
1 tbs. ground flax or hulled hemp hearts
Calories: 624, Protein: 7.9g, Fat 54.5g, Carbs: 36.1g,
Vit. A: 3%, Vit C: 68%, Calcium: 8%, Iron: 26%

Chocolate Avocado Smoothie (serves 2)

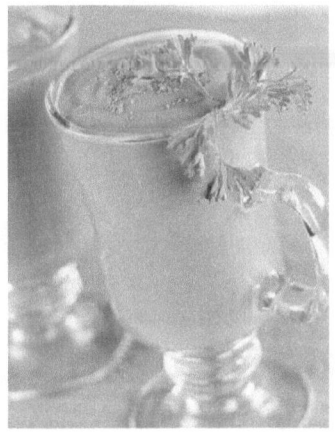

1 avocado
2 frozen bananas
½ cup frozen raspberries (or fresh raspberries or other berries)
1-2 tablespoons unsweetened cocoa powder
2 cups almond or coconut milk
Calories: 930, Protein: 24.3g, Fat 68g, Carbs: 73.8g, Vit. A: 5%, Vit C: 51%, Calcium: 29%, Iron: 29%

Tropical Smoothie (serves 2)

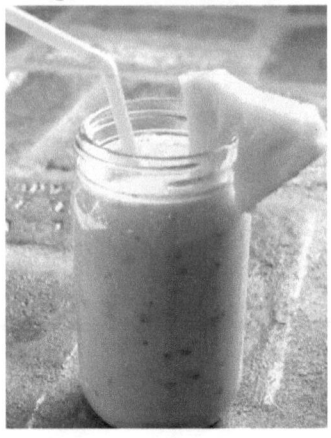

1/4 pineapple, peeled and cubed
1 medium apple, cored and cubed
1 banana, sliced
1 cup almond milk or coconut milk
1 tbsp. 100% mct oil
Calories: 834, Protein: 8.2g, Fat 58g, Carbs: 87g,
Vit. A: 3%, Vit C: 183%, Calcium: 7%, Iron: 31%

Hunger Management Smoothie (serves 2)

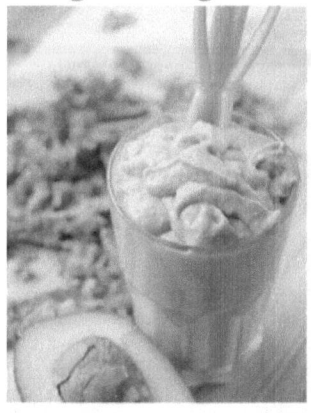

1 banana
1/2 avocado
1-2 tbsp. coconut oil
1/4c coconut milk
1c water
1 tbsp. true or Ceylon cinnamon (or 1 tsp conventional cinnamon)
Calories: 283, Protein: 2.3g, Fat 23.9g, Carbs: 19.5g,
Vit. A: 2%, Vit C: 18%, Calcium: 2%, Iron: 5%

Green Pina Colada Smoothie (serves 2)

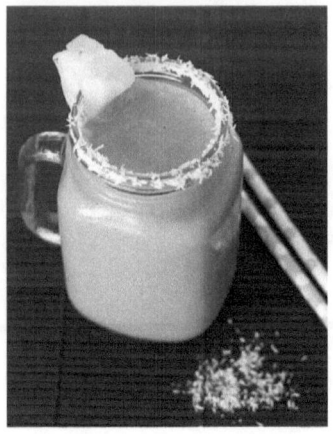

1 cup coconut milk
1 cup spinach, packed
½-frozen banana
1 cup frozen pineapple chunks
Calories: 411, Protein: 4g, Fat 28.9g, Carbs: 41.1g,
Vit. A: 29%, Vit C: 33%, Calcium: 5%, Iron: 16%

Lean Green Smoothie (serves 4)

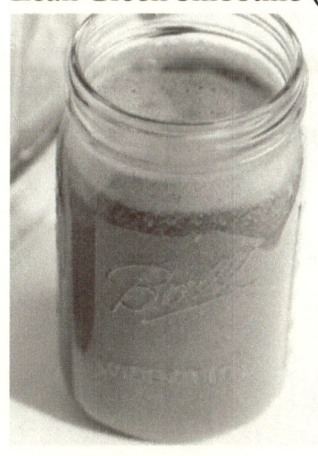

2 oranges, peeled
2 cups pineapple, chopped
6 kale leaves, stalks removed
2 cups mango kombucha
2 cups water
Calories: 104, Protein: 1.3g, Fat 0.2g, Carbs: 26.6g,
Vit. A: 5%, Vit C: 147%, Calcium: 5%, Iron: 2%

Paleo Orange Greensicle Smoothie - A Full Meal Deal!

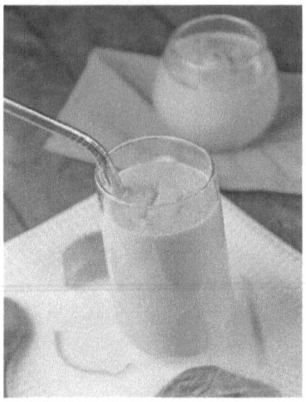

2 cups Unsweetened Coconut Milk
2 navel orange, zested, and peeled with a knife
2 handful baby greens
¼ cup raw cashews
2 tablespoons coconut butter or oil
½ cup frozen mango (or fresh with some ice)
Liquid stevia to taste
Calories: 835, Protein: 10.7g, Fat 74.7g, Carbs: 44.1g, Vit. A: 8%, Vit C: 175%, Calcium: 12%, Iron: 31%

Sunrise Green Smoothie (serves 1)

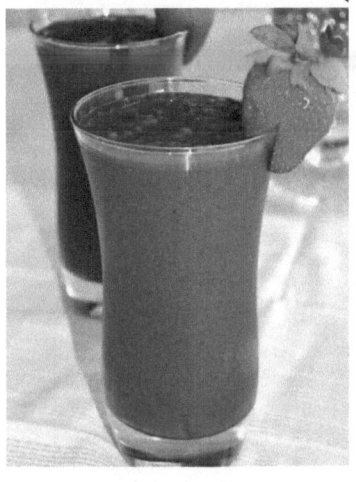

½ Banana, frozen
1 cup Blueberries, frozen
2 cups Spinach
1 cup Strawberries, frozen
1 cup Vanilla almond milk, unsweetened
2 tbsp.   Flax seeds
Calories: 299, Protein: 8g, Fat 8.2g, Carbs: 52.7g,
Vit. A: 124%, Vit C: 216%, Calcium: 54%, Iron:
51%

Orange Green Smoothie (serves 2)

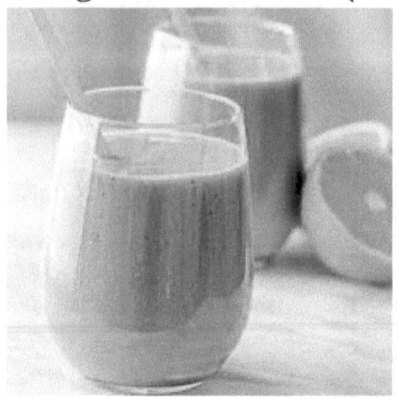

1 Banana
1 Orange
1 1/2 cups Pineapple, frozen
2 cups Spinach, fresh
1 cup Coconut milk, unsweetened
2 tsp Chia seeds
Calories: 596, Protein: 12g, Fat 38.8g, Carbs: 58.8g,
Vit. A: 63%, Vit C: 208%, Calcium: 40%, Iron:
44%

Fruit-Free Green Smoothie (serves 1)

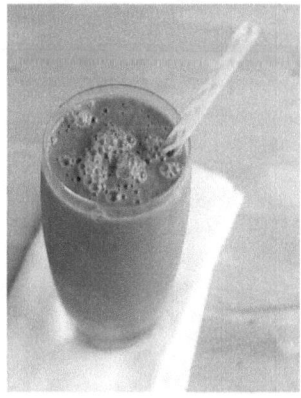

½ organic cucumber, chopped
¼ cup parsley
½ lemon, peeled
½ avocado, pitted and peeled
2 cups organic, raw spinach
1 cup coconut water
6 ice cubes
Calories: 292, Protein: 6.8g, Fat 20.6g, Carbs: 26.1g,
Vit. A: 144%, Vit C: 95%, Calcium: 17%, Iron:
24%

Superfood Chia Green Smoothie Recipe (serves 2)

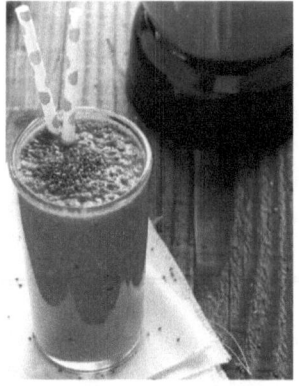

2 cups cold water
2 handfuls spinach
1 kale leaf, medium
1/2 long English cucumber, sliced
1/2 any apple, chopped and not cored/seeded/peeled
2 tbsp. chia seeds
1/2 lemon, juice of
Calories: 42, Protein: 1.5g, Fat 0.3g, Carbs: 10.1g,
Vit. A: 58%, Vit C: 23%, Calcium: 5%, Iron: 7%

Minty Morning Green Smoothie (serves 1)

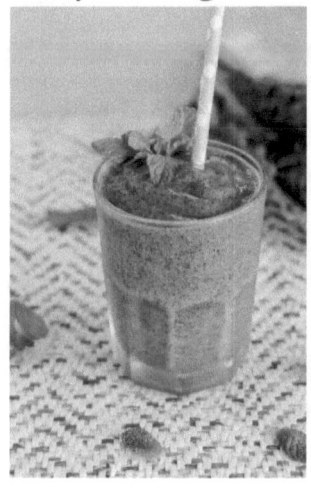

½ Avocado, small
1 cup Baby spinach
½ Banana, frozen
1 tbsp.   Mint, fresh
½ Zucchini or cucumber, raw
1/2 cup Coconut milk
1 Honey or stevia to sweeten
½ Lemon juice, squeezed
1 Dash   Cinnamon
1/2 cup Water
Calories: 306, Protein: 4.8g, Fat 22.4g, Carbs: 28.2g,
Vit. A: 74%, Vit C: 68%, Calcium: 12%, Iron: 17%

Metabolism Booster Smoothie (1 serving)

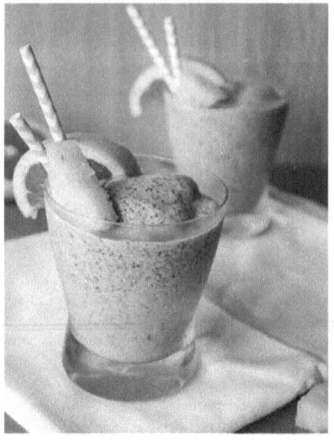

1 Banana, unripe
1 Grapefruit, large
1/2 cup Green tea, strong
1 cup Pineapple, frozen
70 g Spinach
1/4 cup Coconut milk
10 g Whey protein, plain
4 Ice cubes, large
Calories: 877, Protein: 25g, Fat 59g, Carbs: 77g, Vit.
A: 83%, Vit C: 247%, Calcium: 21%, Iron: 35%

Wake Me Up, Keep Me Going Smoothie (serves 2)

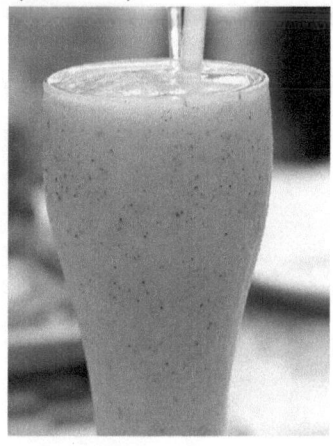

½ Avocado
1 Banana, frozen
1/2 cup Grapes of any color, frozen
1 1/2 cups Green tea
1 cup Kale
1 cup Spinach, loosely packed
Calories: 310, Protein: 3.2g, Fat 20g, Carbs: 35.6g,
Vit. A: 4%, Vit C: 34%, Calcium: 2%, Iron: 5%

Green Detox Juice (Serves 1)

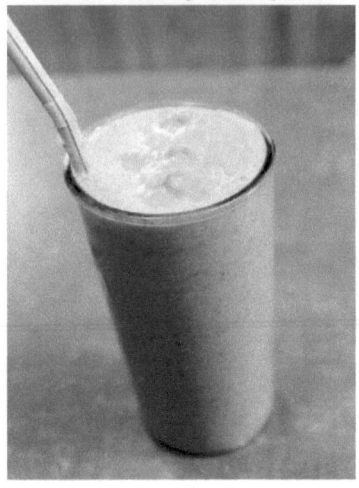

1 Handful of Parsley
1 Handful of cilantro
2 carrots
1 apple, seeded
3 celery ribs
One inch slice of ginger
½ beet with green top
Calories: 145, Protein: 1.5g, Fat 0.3g, Carbs: 37.1g,
   Vit. A: 408%, Vit C: 35%, Calcium: 4%, Iron: 7%

Basic Vegetable Juice (Serves 1)

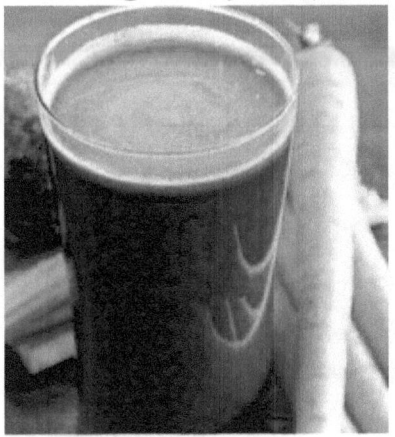

1 Beet
3 Carrots
1 Apple
A bunch of kale
4 Celery sticks
Calories: 214, Protein: 3.7g, Fat 0.5g, Carbs: 53.1g,
Vit. A: 612%, Vit C: 47%, Calcium: 8%, Iron: 12%

Ginger Citrus Juice (serves 1)

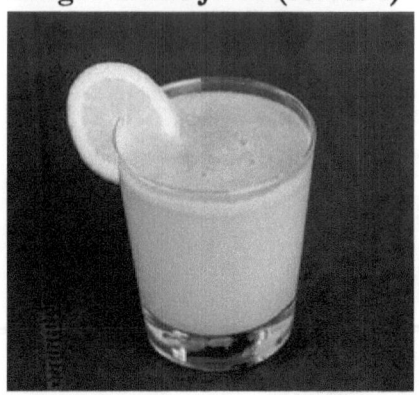

1 Sweet Potato
4 Celery Sticks
1 Inch Ginger
1 Peeled Orange
Calories: 205, Protein: 4g, Fat 0.4g, Carbs: 48.4g,
Vit. A: 17%, Vit C: 225%, Calcium: 8%, Iron: 23%

Parsnip Pear Juice (serves 1)

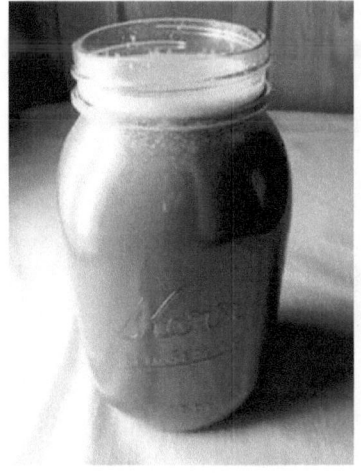

2 parsnips
2 Pears
4 Celery Stalks
1 Cucumber
Calories: 398, Protein: 5.5g, Fat 1.4g, Carbs: 100.5g,
Vit. A: 15%, Vit C: 85%, Calcium: 16%, Iron: 14%

Berry Juice (serves 1)

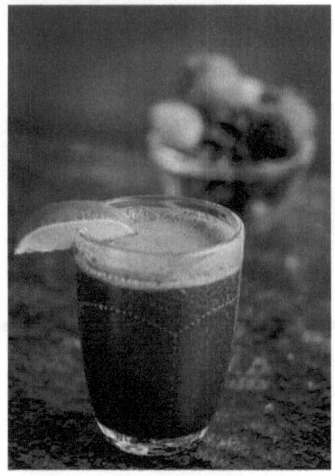

1 Pack Blueberries
1 Pack Blackberries
2 Cups Strawberries
1 Lime
Calories: 340, Protein: 7.3g, Fat 2.9g, Carbs: 83.9g,
  Vit. A: 11%, Vit C: 454%, Calcium: 14%, Iron:
  34%

Paleo Green Smoothie Recipe (serves 2)

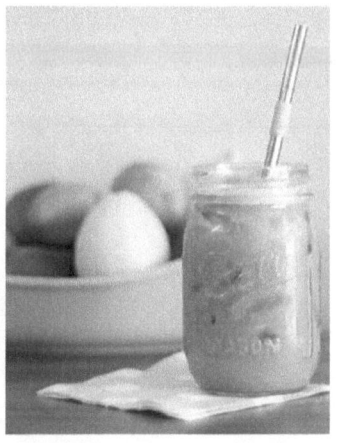

1 1/2 cups coconut water
1/2 cup coconut milk
2 TBS ground flax seed
Juice of one small lemon (or 1/2 large lemon)
1/2 apple (roughly chopped, seeds and core removed) OR 1 pear (roughly chopped, seeds removed)
1/2 orange (peeled, roughly chopped)
3 stalks of celery (roughly chopped)
4 large kale leaves (ribs removed)
6 romaine lettuce leaves
Calories: 282, Protein: 6g, Fat 17.1g, Carbs: 29.3g, Vit. A: 135%, Vit C: 144%, Calcium: 14%, Iron: 27%

Green Machine Smoothie (serves 1)

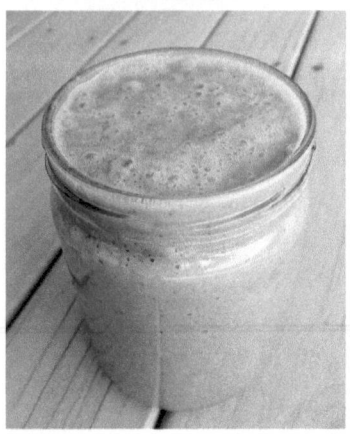

1 Cup Coconut Milk
1/2 Banana
Handful of Spinach
1/2 Avocado
Coconut Water (pour enough in to make the
smoothie have a good balance of liquids and
solids)
Calories: 849, Protein: 9.5g, Fat 77.4g, Carbs: 43.1g,
Vit. A: 4%, Vit C: 45%, Calcium: 10%, Iron: 29%

Almond Avocado Smoothie (serves 1)

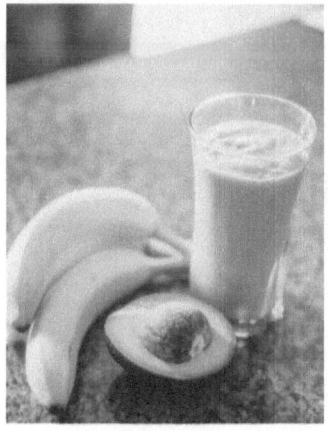

1 cup almond milk
¼ cup blanched almonds
½ small banana
5 tbsp. avocado
¼ cup ice
Calories: 827, Protein: 11.9g, Fat 78.2g, Carbs:
33.8g, Vit. A: 2%, Vit C: 26%, Calcium: 11%, Iron:
29%

Kale Green Fruit Smoothie (serves 2)

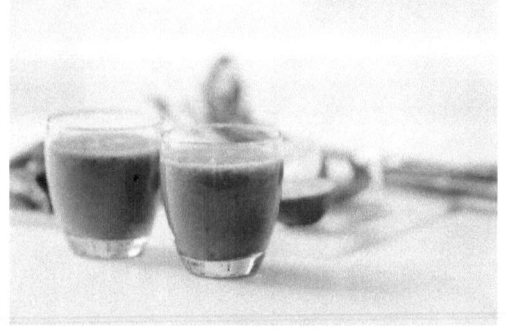

1½ cup coconut water
½ cup coconut milk
4 large Kale leaves, with ribs removed
3 stalks celery
6 leaves romaine lettuce
½ orange, peeled
½ apple, quartered and cored or 1 pear, quartered and cored
3 tbsp. lemon juice
2 tbsp. ground flax seed
Calories: 287, Protein: 6.2g, Fat 17.2g, Carbs: 29.8g, Vit. A: 135%, Vit C: 162%, Calcium: 14%, Iron: 27%

Breakfast Smoothie (serves 2)

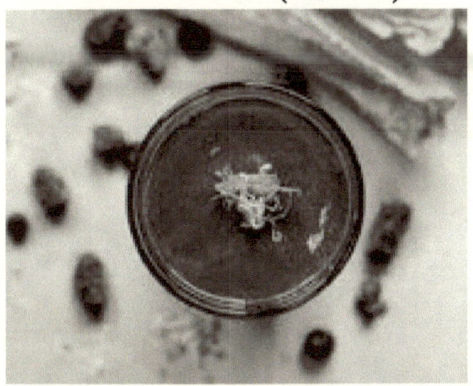

1 cup coconut water
½ cup coconut milk
½ cup frozen blueberries
1 cup frozen blackberries
1 tbsp. chia seeds
2 tbsp. flax powder
Blend together all ingredients except of the chia seeds until the smoothie reaches the desired consistency. Then add seeds.
Calories: 381, Protein: 9.7g, Fat 19.8g, Carbs: 30.2g, Vit. A: 3%, Vit C: 48%, Calcium: 25%, Iron: 31%

Tomato Smoothie (serves 1)

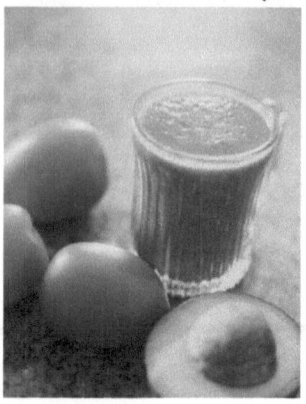

½ chopped tomato
¼ chopped cucumber
½ cup avocado
⅓ cup spinach
1 tsp your favorite hot sauce
A squeeze of lemon
½ c ice
Calories: 172, Protein: 2.7g, Fat 14.5g, Carbs: 11.2g,
Vit. A: 37%, Vit C: 45%, Calcium: 3%, Iron: 6%

Lemon Lime Cucumber Smoothie (serves 1)

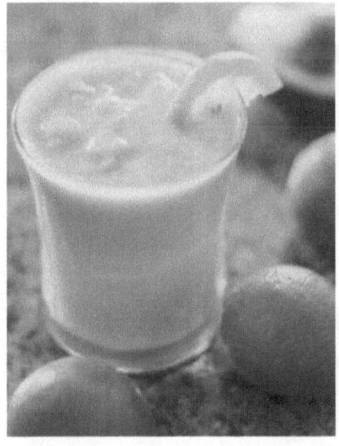

1 tbsp. lemon juice
1 tbsp. lime juice
4/5 c or 7 oz. cucumber, peeled
1 tbsp. avocado
2 pinches sea salt
2 pinches black pepper
¼ cup ice
Calories: 53, Protein: 1.6g, Fat 2.1g, Carbs: 8.4g,
Vit. A: 5%, Vit C: 23%, Calcium: 3%, Iron: 4%

Tropical Mango-Carrot with Pineapple Smoothie (serves 1)

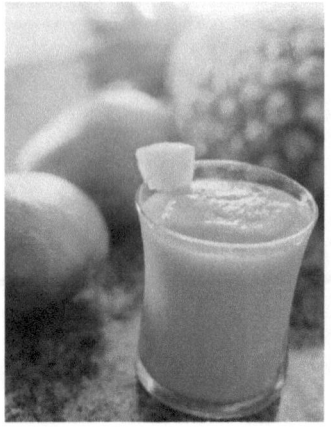

8 oz. filtered water
1 large mango, peeled and pitted
1 medium carrot
¼ c pineapple, diced
Calories: 190, Protein: 1.8g, Fat 0.6g, Carbs: 46.6g,
Vit. A: 236%, Vit C: 134%, Calcium: 5%, Iron: 3%

In the following recipes, you can substitute the water for coconut water, coconut milk, or almond milk. This will add more protein to your smoothie. They are all single serving recipes. The nutrition information offered here is for when these smoothies are made with water.

Exotic Juice

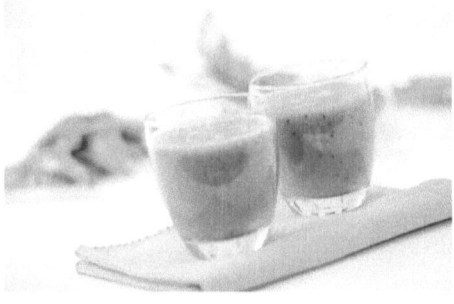

2 cups Water
1 Mango
1 cup Pineapple
1 cup mixed baby leaves
1 tbsp. chia seeds
Calories: 243, Protein: 4.2g, Fat 1.1g, Carbs: 57.3g,
Vit. A: 34%, Vit C: 227%, Calcium: 6%, Iron: 4%

Raspberry Ripple

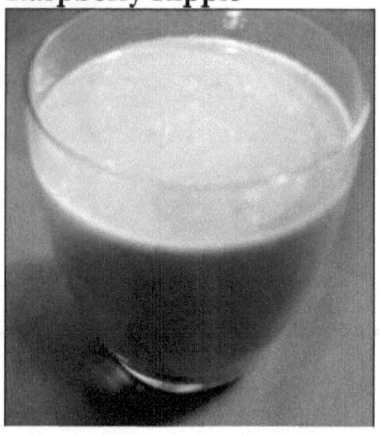

2 Cups Water
1 cup Raspberries
1 Banana
1 cup Bok choy/Pak Choi
Calories: 179, Protein: 3.8g, Fat 1.2g, Carbs: 43.6g,
Vit. A: 42%, Vit C: 121%, Calcium: 13%, Iron:
10%

Crazy Coconut Juice

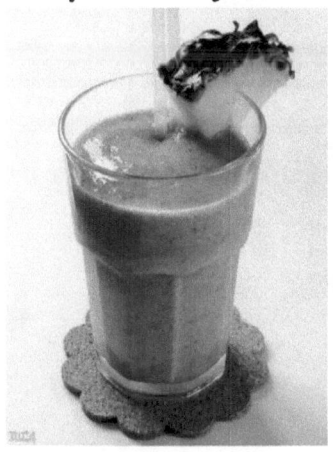

1 cup Water
1 Pineapple
½ cup Coconut
1 cup Spinach
Calories: 231, Protein: 3.1g, Fat 13.7g, Carbs: 28.8g,
Vit. A: 58%, Vit C: 150%, Calcium: 7%, Iron: 38%

Basic Banana

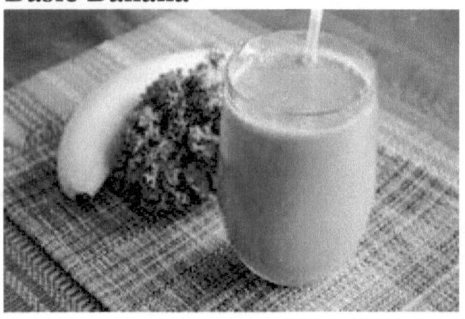

1 cup Water
2 Bananas
1 cup Kale
Calories: 243, Protein: 4.6g, Fat 0.8g, Carbs: 60.9g,
Vit. A: 209%, Vit C: 168%, Calcium: 11%, Iron:
9%

Citrus Cooler

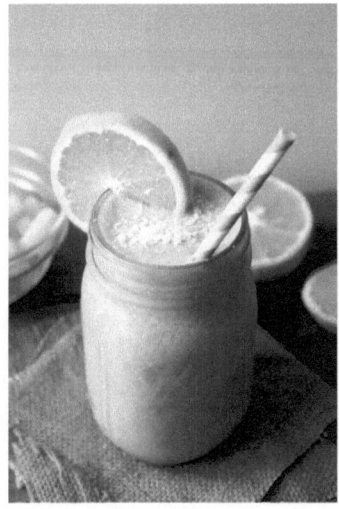

1 cup Water
1 cup Pineapple
1 Orange
1 cup Spinach
Calories: 175, Protein: 3.5g, Fat 0.5g, Carbs: 44.4g,
Vit. A: 66%, Vit C: 309%, Calcium: 13%, Iron: 8%

Sweetness Start

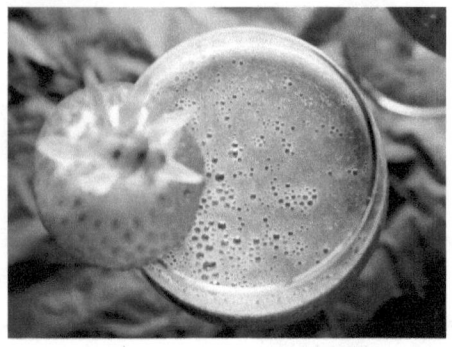

2 cups Water
1 cup Strawberries
1 Mango
1 cup Spinach
Calories: 198, Protein: 2.9g, Fat 1.1g, Carbs: 47.4g,
Vit. A: 88%, Vit C: 251%, Calcium: 9%, Iron: 9%

Strawberry Soul

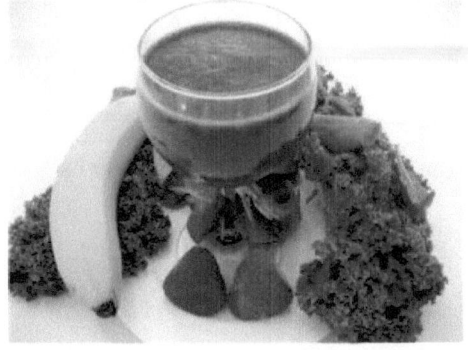

1 cup Water
1 cup Strawberries
1 Banana
1 cup Romaine Lettuce
1 cup of kale leaves, chopped
Calories: 159, Protein: 2.5g, Fat 0.9g, Carbs: 39.7g,
Vit. A: 2%, Vit C: 162%, Calcium: 4%, Iron: 13%

Conclusion:

With the many and varied health benefits of smoothies and juicing, there is no reason not to start now. Even replacing one meal or snack with a smoothie will increase your health. You can lose weight, have more energy, and protect your body from the ravages of disease and aging. All the recipes contained here are delicious and nutritious and you'll love to drink them. And you'll feel great! In the end, isn't that what it's all about?

Thanks again for reading. Here's to a healthier you!

Also, don't forget to grab our free weight loss report to maximize your chances of success at **flatbellyqueens.com**

Finally, if you enjoyed this book, then I'd like to ask you for a favor: would you be kind enough to leave a review for this book on Amazon? It'd be greatly appreciated!

Thank you and good luck!

You may also like these books

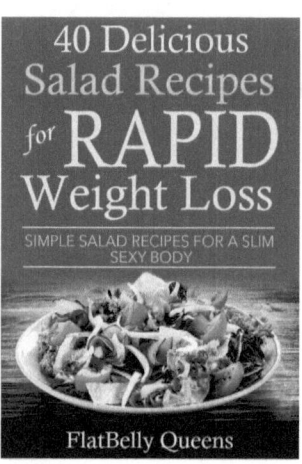

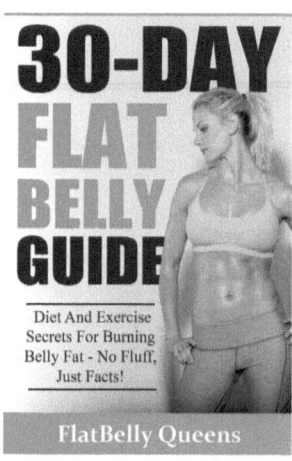

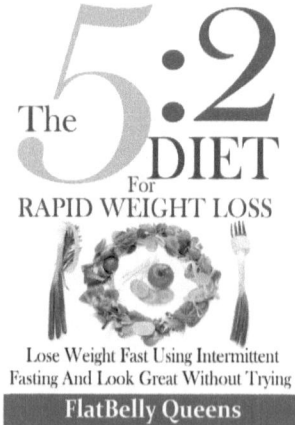

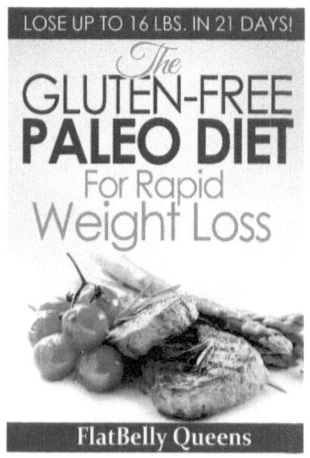